COVID-19:
60 LESSONS LEARNT
ABOUT LIFE AND
OURSELVES
(AUS AND USA)

Covid-19: 60 Lessons Learnt About Life And Ourselves (AUS and USA)

A survey of AUS and USA residents

GLENNYS MARSDON

Zeitgeist Creations

Praise for the author's writing

Contents

Covid-19 the bug that crashed
uninvited into our lives and refused to
leave until we'd learnt our lesson. But
exactly what lessons did we learn?

Immense thanks goes out to all the
essential workers who repeatedly put
their lives on the line for us.

Introduction

There is nothing funny about the Corona Virus (Covid-19). As one West Australian recently said ...

"It's cruel, tough and in some cases deadly."

My heart goes out to anyone who has lost a loved one. Having lost a partner myself in sudden circumstances some years back, I cannot begin to fathom what your loss must be like during times of isolation and restrictive funerals. I wish you all well on the journey.

Being a freelancer who has lost all six of my income streams overnight, I have some idea of the impact of Covid-19 on my fellow unemployed. My thoughts go out to anyone who has lost a business they've taken years to build.

In some small attempt to make these losses meaningful, I think it's important to consider what we've learnt during this period. In just six weeks we have learnt so much about life in general and ourselves.

So, what have we learnt?

As is our want at *The Ponder Room*, we sat and had a big ponder about the lessons learnt. To supplement this, we conducted a short feedback exercise amongst 55 **West Australian residents** between April 20th and 27th.

We also tapped into another survey undertaken by professional research company *Thinkfield*. Conducted in

April the *Thinkfield* survey sought the opinions of 276 West Australians.

The American survey was based on a random sample of 122 **residents of America.** It was conducted during the last week of April 2020.

The American sample included a good spread of age groups with one third aged 18-29 years (33%), one third 30-44 (30%), nearly one third 45-60 (27%) and one in ten over 60 years (10%). The final sample was slightly skewed towards females (60%).

Thank you to anyone who took part in either of these surveys. Keep safe, well, and watch out for more informal surveys on topics of interest.

Glennys

Section A: Western Australian Survey

Chapter 1

Personal impact of Covid (WA)

An online survey of 276 West Australians was conducted by Western Australian professional research company *Thinkfield* during the first week of April 2020. In addition a feedback exercise was undertaken on our consumer psychology blog called *The Ponder Room*. Following is a combination of these findings.

Interest in life in general

Respondents in the *Thinkfield* survey were asked how they felt about life in general using a 10 point scale where 10 was "terrific" and 1 was "not wanting to get out of bed and take part in life".

The vast majority (88%) of West Australian respondents showed a positive outlook towards life.

For example:

- One in two (56%) picked a score of 7 or more;
- One in three (32%) scored themselves a mid-level 5 or 6;
- Meanwhile one in ten (13%) rated a 1-3, meaning they were less interested in life.

Areas of Impact

In *The Ponder Room* feedback exercise some 55 West Australian respondents were shown a list of five areas and asked whether they had been impacted in each area.

The five areas under review were:

Work
Social
Exercise
Dietary
Personal development

The results have been presented in this section.

Social Life

As March turned into April West Australian residents were told to bunker down at home. The only exemption was people working in essential services. For the rest of us we could only venture out for medical appointments, to shop, exercise or go to work. It's hardly surprising then that social life was nominated as the main area of impact.

During the *Thinkfield* survey, three in five respondents (57%) said they were either "extremely" or "very" keen to keep in touch with other people, so they didn't become socially isolated. A further one third (30%) were moderately interested in doing so. Meanwhile, one in ten were slightly keen (11%) and 2% were not at all keen.

In *The Ponder Room* feedback exercise, one in five respondents said they had indeed been more social during isolation, whereas one in ten had been less social.

The results imply that somehow being told to socially isolate had made people more social. Specifically, they were more likely to have talked to family and friends. Anyone who has a Facebook or Instagram can attest to the flood of notifications from friends and family. So too anyone who has participated in a Zoom, Skype, Messenger or Facebook Teams meeting.

Indeed, amongst the *Thinkfield* respondents:

- ◦ One in two (54%) had talked to someone via a video link up during April. In addition, one in ten (8%) had been involved in an online group meeting;
- ◦ One third had either visited someone at home or had someone visit them at home (39%);

- One in six (16%) had met someone in a public venue e.g. park or shops;
- One in ten (8%) had chatted to a neighbour over the fence;
- One in ten (10%) had heard from someone they hadn't heard from in a long time;
- Only 2% or less had written a card to someone.
- The same proportion had either: undertaken or received a drive by toot; shared something they'd stocked up on; or given/received muffins or a meal.

Exercise

In our weight loss obsessed society, many people had exercise on their "to do" list. With fewer distractions things started off well for the many. However, some of us went into a panic mode. Would everyone emerge from this time as six-packed ripped Adonis's? Would we be the odd man (or woman) out. Would our sloth be accentuated?

Then the gyms were closed, and we sloths were saved. Or so we thought.

Parks became festooned with lycra, yoga mats and dumbbells. Personal trainers were in high demand.

As the number of new Covid-19 cases continued to rise, more restrictions were put in place. Outdoor exercise groups were soon limited to one or two people including the trainer. But people wouldn't be held back, they started walking.

Results from The Ponder Room exercise showed that one in six respondents were exercising more. On the other hand, one in seven had been exercising less.

Perhaps the equilibrium would be maintained, and we'd be blend in okay.

Work

Much has been written about the impact of Covid-19 on livelihoods, the constant balancing act between health and wealth.

I've lost count of the number of people I know who've had their workload not just reduced but vanish altogether. My friends working in the creative and entertainment industries have been severely hit. They are a robust crew who have reinvented themselves many times over, but this one has really knocked them for six.

The Ponder Room exercise revealed that one in seven respondents had lost work. This echoes the unemployment figure of around 10%.

Interestingly, that same exercise revealed that one in twenty respondents had actually gained work.

Dietary habits

It wasn't long before entertainment venues shut up shop. Some valiantly tried to stay open by only selling every second seat, however this only lasted a week before they closed up too. What to do?

Television became a central escape.

And so, it was that those of us without Netflix, Stan or any of the other streaming services, sat down to watch MasterChef and Jamie Oliver's latest offering. It wasn't long before the direct relationship between boredom and trips to the fridge kicked in.

As restaurants closed some people attempted to channel Jamie Oliver. Given the number of bike food couriers on the empty city streets, it would seem that many people resorted to delivery services. At one point, food bike couriers were the only other people on the streets, besides the police and council security cars.

The Ponder Room exercise suggested that one in ten respondents were eating less healthy. Meanwhile one in twenty reported eating healthier. I bet they have personal trainers too.

Personal development

As the lock-down took hold people eagerly professed their intent to improve themselves. Learning a new skill, language or being more creative were common goals. Social media heard their cries and responded.

Online courses invaded social media, with ads popping up every half hour. Most of the ads promised amazing results from free offerings. However, on further inspection the "free" component had little value other than as a lead generator for the author, with a secondary suggestion that the reader spend $200 on the real course.

After six weeks it was clear that reality was different. By mid-April only one in twenty respondents in *The Ponder*

Room exercise had undertaken some kind of personal development.

Other impacts

Respondents were asked to make any other comments about how they'd been impacted. The following two comments sum up the extremes of respondents' experiences.

"I'm more relaxed than usual, almost like a holiday."

"I'm being less social i.e. talking less to friends/family. Doing less exercise. Eating less healthy meals. I've lost work. I work from home, alone, or at least I did. My quiet office with fast internet is now a noisy place full of other people teleconferencing, learning, interrupting me, while the internet drops out periodically with no warning, accompanied by loud complaints from everyone else, making it impossible for me to do my job."

Chapter 2

Lessons learnt about life (WA)

Respondents were asked what lessons they had learnt about life in general. Their answers fell into 23 areas as presented in this section.

Heroes redefined

One of the biggest lessons, mentioned by several respondents, was learning who the true heroes are.

Not superstars
Not sportspeople
Not billionaires

Although thanks does have to go to Twiggy Forrest who managed to secure much needed Personal Protection Equipment.

The true heroes were those working in essential services, particularly the health system. Those who thought beyond their own lives and families. Who risked their own lives over and over again, to provide essential services while we ran away and hid.

> *"I can't imagine how they do it. I know it is their job but really. And some have moved away from their family too, they are the heroes in this."*

Not taking life for granted

Another frequently made comment was about not taking life for granted. This included the realisation that "life is short", "fragile" and can change in an instant.

Consequently, there were several comments about "making the most of" or "valuing every day" and every moment.

It followed that some mention making sure you have your priorities in order.

> *"Never take the future for granted, life can change significantly in the blink of an eye and there is nothing you can do to prevent it happening."*

> *"To keep your priorities straight, life is too short and too fragile. Never take anything for granted."*

Improved community spirit

Several respondents spoke about a more positive community spirit. That people were more likely to say hello to each other and smile. One respondent mentioned "a pandemic of kindness".

Having said this it was conceded that difficult times bringing out both the best and worst in people.

> *"That we have great community spirit in Perth."*

> *"How kind people are when things get tough. I believe there is a pandemic of kindness running in parallel with Covid-19."*

Little things mean a lot

Talking about community spirit. It was surprising how quickly people started looking out for their fellow man. The media reported an avalanche of good news stories.

In most instances these random acts of kindness were small gestures not sumptuous offerings. e.g. people offering to pick up grocery items.

> *"While I was down the shops, I rang my neighbours to see if they wanted anything, I've never done that before. They were so thankful."*

> *"I overheard a conversation where the lady was explaining that she'd had to flee her home, she couldn't*

go back. While she was talking she was trying to look after a toddler and a baby in a pram. This other lady, a stranger, came over and gave her a bucket of hot chips to keep the toddler quiet. At first she didn't want to accept it, but in the end she did."

Looking after the vulnerable

This sentiment of helping others was also seen in a program called *Hotels with Heart*. Held at the Pan Pacific Hotel in Perth, the one-month trial saw 20 homeless people isolate inside. There they enjoyed a shower, clean clothes and a bed for the quarantine period. It will be interesting to see what long term impact this has on their lives. To date there have been no negatives reported publicly about this initiative, from either side.

In contrast, some of the cruise ship passengers who were also put up at 5-star hotels (at the governments expense), complained about the conditions and the food, with a few even throwing their meals over the balconies.

"Many people experiencing homelessness have chronic health and mental health issues. The 'Hotels With Heart' pilot learns from similar initiatives happening around the world," said Community Services Minister Simone McGurk.

Live with less

In *The Ponder Room* exercise several respondents said they'd learnt that they could live with less.

"We don't actually need much to survive."

"You can live with a lot less things."

"We can survive with a few basic things."

Slowing down

Similarly, comments were made about getting off the fast-paced treadmill and learning to slow down. One respondent was surprised that slowing down can be a "guilt free" experience.

Other respondents were surprised by the benefits of slowing down.

"There are many things to gain by slowing down."

"Slowing down really can be a guilt free experience."

Essentials redefined

Early on Covid-19 raised the issue of what constitutes essential services and essential trips. This generated considerable debate.

In the end essential reasons for being outdoors were defined as: medical appointments, going to the chemists, grocery shopping, exercise, and going to work.

Meanwhile essential services were identified as: medical, school, hair dressing, transport, chemists and supermarkets.

So now we all know where we fit in the scheme of things.

Thankfully the idea of a 30 minute haircut lasted as long as it took for policy-makers to go home and tell their partners.

Queuing

With cafes limited to takeaway, and supermarkets worried about contamination, the world of shopping was soon marked out with social distancing measures.

The public soon learnt how to stand behind the line or on the 'x' marking the spot.

Consumer behaviour changed overnight. Our ability to wait patiently was in stark contrast to the usual Boxing Day sales or early Covid-19 toilet roll war.

A few respondents in *The Ponder Room* exercise commented about how the public learnt to be patient and even got on well when waiting in queues.

"Who'd have thought we knew how to wait politely? That would not have happened a year ago. We seem more patient."

Shopping hygiene

While talking about shopping, our eyes were opened to the potential health hazards in shopping centres, cafes, and restaurants.

The main focus was on shopping trolleys, something we'd never considered before. Another casualty in the cleanliness war was the communal newspaper or magazine. Some cafes also alerted us to the perils of using shared cutlery.

"The way they panicked about shopping trolleys I think I'm going to keep wearing gloves after this."

"My favourite café introduced single-use cutlery instead of the usual ones. I've never thought about this before."

"At my fish supplier customers have to sanitise their hands and wear plastic gloves."

Supply and Demand

Petrol and toilet rolls provided a basic lesson in supply and demand. Consumers were reminded of their power.

Petrol prices reduced to an all-time low as the public put their cars in the garage and bunker-ed down.

Meanwhile the price of toilet rolls went through the roof on eBay as hoarders tried to capitalise on the lack of supply. Thankfully, this was soon nipped in the bud, with people being identified and fined.

"We aren't using our cars as much, so the price of petrol goes down."

Social Media for good

In the years leading up to Covid-19, social media coped a hammering for its negative sides of bullying and trolls. Strangely, the incidence of these actions appeared to fade away.

Hopefully, this was a real change. Or maybe it was just a case of the phenomenon not being able to get as much airtime.

Instead social media was heralded as being used for good, not evil e.g. online meetings, gym sessions, social catch-ups, and family challenges.

"We used Zoom to catch up with friends overseas, it was so good to see them."

"The family challenges on Tik Tok are loads of fun."

Business Pivoting

Prior to Covid-19 whenever I heard the word 'pivot' I'd think back to ballet lessons. Either that or a cumbersome Excel pivot table, which if you have ever experienced one, you know not to invite it back into your life any time soon.

Through Covid-19 we learnt about nimble businesses that were thinking outside the square and pivoting their structure into new areas. Sure, the restructuring was in their interests as it helped their bottom line, but the changes also helped society.

Fashion designers started making medical tunics and masks, which let's be honest wasn't too much of a stretch. Praise goes to the whisky distiller who started making hand sanitiser.

> *"That whiskey place was a good idea, but I hope they wash the vats well when they go back to making whiskey."*

The Environment

Several respondents mentioned the positive impact of Covid-19 on the environment.

With fewer cars on the roads the air quality improved in many countries. No doubt the same can be said for Perth, although the change is less visible with our clear blue skies.

"How humans are stuffing up the world and how nature fixes it when we are not there."

"The animals are starting to reclaim the towns overseas ... it makes you wonder doesn't it?"

"I heard that in Adelaide kangaroos were in the city."

Natural penicillin

Recent years has seen an increasing focus on green medicine. More and more health professional talk about the benefits of getting out into nature, be it a walk in the park or quick dip in the sea.

Thanks to Covid-19 people were reminded of the joys of being out in nature. Parks were dotted with groups of one or two people walking in sunshine and getting back to nature.

Cycle paths were like freeways, as bike shops struggled to keep up with demand.

"Seeing all the people in the parks, all the families out playing, throwing Frisbees, kick footballs, it's great."

Social distancing

While people embraced the outdoors, we also learnt about social distancing and the health benefits of keeping 1.5 metres apart.

Two respondents in *The Ponder Room* exercise had been surprised to read about how far sweat propels off joggers. This had them rethinking where they go walking.

> *"I never knew how far the sweat goes when people run past me. That's something to think about when I go for a run."*

Fighting spirit of the elderly

A couple of comments were made about the elderly being told they would "not be resuscitated" if they contracted Covid-19 and ended up requiring ventilation. Some respondents felt the elderly did not need to hear this. Others said more thought should be given to how this message was communicated.

At the same time there were also comments made about Captain Thomas Moore who at 99 years young completed over 100 laps of his backyard to raise money for the NHS. On the day of his 100th birthday he'd raised over 32 million pounds.

> *"What a comment to hear, that my Aunty will be left to die. Why should she bother anymore? She's worked so hard for years to stay alive. When she heard this, she went into a bit of a depression."*

> *"Look at Captain Moore. We shouldn't write them off just because of their age."*

Politicians can work together

Several respondents mentioned the sheer delight of seeing politicians working together to solve a common problem.

Several said it was a relief, others said it provided a good role model for children.

> *"Who knew they could work in harmony on an issue, shame it took a worldwide pandemic to make it happen."*

> *"So good for my boys to see our top leaders working together on a problem."*

> *"I like not seeing them all just yelling at each other in parliament. Would be nice not to have to see that again."*

Weddings redefined

The wedding industry accounts for millions of dollars and much agony for those who have ever had to plan one. The venue hire, food, drinks, dresses, suits, guest gifts and on and on, before you add in the honeymoon.

Through Covid-19 people learnt they could get married without having to rack up a huge debt.

> *"Instead of all the fancy stuff, which is just to show off to others really, we had a house deposit."*

> *"You realise you don't really need all the extras. We can*

*go on a holiday later without the travel agent stinging
us for a honeymoon prices."*

Cruise Ships

In early March our thoughts went out the family and friends of Mr James Kwan, a pioneer of the WA tourism industry, and the first Covid19 passing in Perth. Mr Kwan had seen out his last days on a cruise ship.

As the days and week progressed more cruise ships circled Western Australian waters, each one making Perth residents hold their breath a little tighter. The Artania was particularly worrying with 79 crew and passengers testing positive for Covid19.

Let's be honest, the perceptions of cruise ships took a big hit thanks to Covid-19.

"I'd rethink going on a cruise any time soon."

Teachers and Home schooling

The Western Australian school holidays occurred at the height of Covid19's appearance in Perth. Considerable debate was held about whether to keep children at home or send them back to school. Part of this debate was about parents who worked in essential service areas.

In the end parents (other than essential service workers) were asked to home-school their children.

Consequently, many parents said they gained a whole new appreciation for teachers.

"I learnt teachers deserve the long break."

Importance of family and friends

A small number of respondents voiced a sentiment no doubt felt by a lot of people. They had been reminded about the importance of family and friends.

This included looking beyond their immediate family to make sure others were okay.

"The importance of protecting your health and those close to you."

One world

Covid-19 also highlighted the interconnected world we live in. This was emphasised by the rapid spread of the disease across countries as we become more global citizens.

The experience also highlighted the need to work together as one world to fight a common foe.

"Literally it's a case of if one country coughs another sneezes."

"We can achieve amazing things by working together."

"Hands across the ocean working together was great to see."

Chapter 3

Lessons learnt about ourselves (WA)

Respondents were asked what they had learnt about themselves. Their answers fell into 17 categories.

Resilient, adaptable

Many respondents talked about learning a valuable and pleasing lesson about themselves. The most frequent comment was learning they were much stronger than they thought.

This included being more "resilient", "positive" and "adaptable" than they thought they were.

"That I am resilient and positive."

"How I'm more adaptable than I thought I was."

"That I always look for the positive in situations."

"I'm more vigilant about myself and less careless than I had realised."

"Damn I'm good."

Need external motivation

The second most frequent comment centred on the realisation that they needed external motivation.

This could take the form of definite structure and just a need to be busy.

"I need structure."

"I do less when I have more time."

"I can be really lazy if I don't have external motivation."

Need people/ The value of friends

Similarly, some respondents gained a greater appreciation of their friends.

Others spoke about learning who their true friends were. They now knew who would offer help in times of crisis. Just as importantly, some were surprised who they didn't hear from.

"It has reminded me that I am an extrovert in the true sense of being energised by spending time with people."

"Just how much I value my friends."

"The people who offered help weren't the ones I expected. They were not my closest friends at all."

Family

It was interesting, and a little sad, to hear several respondents talk about reacquainting themselves with their family.

This was particularly so, but certainly not confined to, relatives living overseas.

Thanks to the latest, easy to use, online group platforms, family linkups were conducted more often.

"I like my family better than I thought."

"I like the company of my immediate family."

"I surprised myself. On the first day of isolation I decided I'd be kind to my husband and other people. So far we are in our sixth week and it's working."

Importance of coffee

Another common comment was the importance of coffee. A few respondents were happy to see coffee classed as an essential service.

> *"You can survive anything as long as takeaway coffee is available."*

Life beyond work

Some of the self-reported workaholics reported having a tough time. For some this was because the services they relied on had shut up shop, which meant they were forced to stop work for a while.

Others had difficulty with life encroaching on them whether they wanted it or not. For example, their home-schooling children were only a few steps away.

Either way some of the workaholics learnt there is more to life than working.

> *"My inner drive to work longer and harder stopped for a little bit. I was forced into shut down and after a while I liked it. It was very hard at first though."*

Personal perspective

It follows that some said observing the impact of Covid-19 around the world helped put their own life into perspective.

Reference was made to Italy. Both the impact of the virus and the immense fortitude of the people.

Similarly, the lines of cloaked coffins in New York were deemed hard to fathom, as was the growing death count around the world.

Consequently issues that had trouble them pre-Covid19 seemed trivial.

"You find out what's important in life."

Call a truce

A few respondents said they had reached out to people they had fallen out with. Others had heard from friends they thought were no longer talking to them.

It seems there is nothing like the potential of imminent death to see differences forgotten.

"It seemed silly to not be talking when things were tough. We should be joining together not pulling apart."

"To be honest I couldn't remember what the problem was."

Importance of good hygiene

Several respondents mentioned watching a YouTube video about hand washing.

The video involved someone wearing cream rubber gloves and using a black dye to highlight areas that are often missed.

Others were reminded about the importance of cleaning down surfaces, and the dangers hidden in public surfaces e.g. handrails, doorknobs and traffic light buttons.

"Men learnt how to wash their hands."

Enjoy isolation

A few respondents learnt that they quite liked being in isolation. This included finding a new appreciation of quietness.

"I so love isolation."

"I can find joy in quietness."

Need own space/ Me Time

In contrast to the last point a few respondents commented that having a fuller house made them value their own space more.

"I value my own space and miss it."

"I need to take more ME time."

"The house is way to hectic."

Be prepared

The panic buying combined with the large-scale loss of jobs saw a few respondents comment about the importance of being more prepared.

This included having some savings and not putting all their eggs in one basket.

"Always have a contingency plan or a 'in case of' fund."

Joy of hugging

Much has been said by mental health experts about the importance of touch. Several respondents were crying out for a hug, particularly those living in single households.

Social isolation may be one thing but the inability to hug loved ones not living in your immediate family is another. This is especially so for the elderly who were living in a precarious situation.

"I can't wait to give my parents a hug."

"My grandparents are getting old. I don't want to hug

them and give them something, but what if this is the last time I see them and I haven't been able to hug them."

"It's like Russian Roulette, what if they catch it and I've missed giving them a hug?"

Buying habits

A few respondents said Covid-19 has impacted on future buying habits. This was particularly for large or delayed purchases.

For most this meant not buying trips, or special events in advance.

"For a while I don't think I'll be booking anything long term ...well at least not 6 months in advance, not in this environment."

Personal truths

A few respondents took away some even greater lessons about themselves and how they face the world. Some personal truths.

"I'm vain and materialistic."

"I'm not good at homeschooling."

"If you're looking for anything outside yourself, look for it within."

One day at a time

One of the most common phrases was one we hear often, *'just take one day at a time."*
However, the phrase seemed to take on more gravitas when people said it now.

"The importance of taking life one day at a time and cherishing the moments."

Chapter 4

The WA experience, a quick recap

"Western Australia is doing very well in terms of Australian and world standards," Premier Mark Mc-Gowan (April 2020).

Western Australia has historically worn the tag of "the most isolated capital in the world". While the 'isolation' title has been contested a few times, there is no doubt that we often watch international issues unfolding from a safe distance. Covid19 was different.

As a member of the community, the first signs that Covid19 was going to touch Western Australia began at the end of February, with rumblings about what was happening overseas.

On March 1, the world had seen 83,000 cases with 2,867 deaths, most of those in China. Australia had 25 confirmed cases. Western Australia reported two cases, both cruise ship passengers.

Sadly, the next day it was reported that one of the cruise ship passengers, a pioneer of the WA tourism industry Mr James Kwan, had passed away. The AMA (Australian Medical Association) predicted one in four West Australians may contract the virus.

Five days later, Perth residents were cancelling overseas trips and stocking up on tinned food, pasta, hand sanitiser, Panadol, cold/flu tablets and the soon to be elusive toilet paper. Some residents even drove 150km to Harvey and wiped out the country town's toilet paper supply. At the same time the Catholic Church in Perth removed holy water and banned the drinking of communion wine from the chalice.

By March 11 at least 450 people had presented to the new West Australian Covid Clinics. The clinics had been set up to test people anyone returning from overseas who was feeling unwell. Businesses were starting to feel the pressure with some considering laying off staff. Qantas Chief Executive, Alan Joyce said he would take no salary for three months, as eight A380's "parked up". The Sydney to London flight was routed through Perth instead of Singapore. Public announcements reminded everyone to wash their hands, refrain from touching their faces, and public surfaces such as lift buttons, railings and doorknobs.

March 15 saw travellers being urged to check the *Smart Traveller* site before commencing their trips. The World Health Organisation said it would be "prudent" to delay travel if you were sick, elderly or had chronic diseases.

Meanwhile travel companies advertised discounted holidays e.g. 5-day Broome package for $897 or 4 days in Cairns for $285.

Also on March 15, anyone who arrived in Australia after that date, (and those who thought they might have been in contact with someone with the virus), were asked to "social isolate" usually in local hotels for 14 days. Some were lucky enough to spend this time confined on Rottnest Island. Every night two Transperth buses whistled down Mounts Bay Road under a four car police escort. They were escorting travellers to city hotels.

By March 20, "social distancing" had become part of our vernacular as we stayed 1.5 metres apart. People stopped shaking hands and hugging. We were being asked to work from home if we could and reconsider all non-essential outings. As a result, cafes and restaurants started introducing more cleaning practices, and reduced the amount of seating. Within two days this had moved to no seating as they were confined to takeaway only.

As the weeks progressed government bans took on a more serious tone.

Bans included no "non-essential" gatherings of 500 people or more. Horror of all horrors, this meant no crowds at AFL football games. Some venues like movie theatres thought creatively and only sold every second seat, however this didn't last long, and they soon closed their doors.

Western Australia closed its border to the eastern states. This was quickly followed with a further to lock down of Perth city with other regional areas. The State was divided up into manageable areas. More and more businesses closed their doors as an increasing number of employees worked from home. The public was asked to stay at home and only travel for work, shopping, medical appointments, to go to the chemist or exercise. While travelling around the suburbs was quiet, it was nothing compared with the ghost town appearance of the inner city. Some of the most at-risk homeless people were housed in city hotels.

Anzac Day commemorations were cancelled. Instead in the early hours of the morning there was an outpouring of love from dark driveways and balconies. Families stood in silence. Some clapped. A few had family members who could play the Last Post. In the city you could hear several buglers playing in the distance.

After several days of zero or one new case being reported in Western Australia, on the week of April 27, the State Government started relaxing a few of the restrictions. People were allowed to go out in groups of up to ten people.

By May 8th Western Australia had reported several days of no new cases, and the focus turned to relaxing further restrictions.

By May 14th more people started emerging from their houses. The unusually dry, cool, blue sky autumns days saw people taking advantage of the ability to meet in groups of 20. You could see people having difficulty maintaining the 1.5 metre distance rule.

On the weekend of June 27th Perth was almost back to normal. Restaurants and cafes had opened, along with some nightclubs. Movie theatres screened their first movies in months. Gyms opened their doors for patrons to assess the damage.

The general sentiment amongst West Australians was that we had been extremely lucky. It was a combination of being seeing the magnitude of what had happened overseas and following the advice given to us.

Section B:
American survey

Chapter 5

Personal impact of Covid (USA)

Like the West Australian respondents, the Americans were asked to describe the impact of Covid on their life.

Social Life

Respondents were asked if they had been more or less social since Covid-19 hit. In this instance being "social" included talking to family or friends.

One in two respondents said they had been less social (49%).

Meanwhile nearly one in five had been more social (18%). In Western Australia this was attributed to the increasing number of online contacts (e.g. via Facetime or Zoom calls), I assume it's the same in the USA.

Exercise

In our weight loss obsessed society, many people had exercise on their "to do" list. With fewer distractions things started off well for many. However, some of us went into a panic mode.

Would everyone emerge from this time as six-packed ripped Adonis's?
Would we be the odd man (or woman) out.
Would our sloth be accentuated?

Around one third of the respondents had undertaken less exercise (35%).

Meanwhile one in four (25%) had undertaken more exercise. I bet they had personal trainers too. Perhaps the equilibrium would be maintained, and I'd be able to blend in okay.

Work

Much has been written about the impact of Covid-19 on livelihoods, along with the constant balancing act between health and wealth.

I've lost count of the number of people I know who've had their workload not just reduced but vanish altogether. My friends working in the creative and entertainment industries have been severely hit. They are a robust crew who have reinvented themselves many times over, but this one has really knocked them for six.

Nearly half of those surveyed said they had lost work (44%).

On the other hand, one in six (16%) had actually gained work.

Dietary Habits

With little to do, television became a central escape in our household and it wasn't long before the direct relationship between boredom and trips to the fridge kicked in.

Food delivery bike couriers were the only people on the streets in Western Australia, besides the police and council security cars. Perhaps it was the same in the USA?

Nearly one in three American respondents (29%) reported eating less healthy.

One in five (24%) said they were eating healthier.

Personal Development

As the lock-down took hold, people eagerly professed their intent to improve themselves. Learning a new skill, language or being more creative were common goals. Social media heard their cries and responded.

Online courses invaded social media, with ads popping up every half hour. Most of the ads promised amazing results from free offerings. However, on further inspection the "free" component had little value other than as a lead generator for the author, with a secondary suggestion that the reader spend $200 on the real course.

After six weeks it was clear that reality was different.

By the end of April only one in four respondents (23%) had undertaken some kind of personal development.

Other impacts

Respondents were asked to make any other comments about how they had been impacted. Several comments referred to home-based projects e.g. completing home décor projects; getting ready to downsize; catching up on housework; cleaning out closets.

Some comments related to schooling e.g. home-schooling and virtual schooling.

Other comments included: reading more books; cooking more; gardening; sleeping poorly; staying home more; completing long overdue tasks; and working from home.

"Having kids out of school was a big change for me."

"Working from home is great."

"My student teaching internship was cut short."

Chapter 6

Lessons learnt about life (USA)

Respondents were asked what lessons they had learnt about life in general. Their answers fell into 11 areas.

Not taking life for granted/Life is short

The most frequently comment, nominated by 15% of American respondents, was about not taking life for granted.

Another 5% added that life is short or valuable and 2% spoke about the "value of normal."

Some respondents went further to discuss the importance of "enjoying" or "cherishing" every moment.

> *"It reminds you not to take anything for granted anymore."*

"Life is valuable and we won't ever again take for granted everything we were able to do pre-Covid."

"Life is short, be healthy."

"Appreciate the thing you have in life now."

"Don't take normal for granted."

"People take the world for granted."

Lack of control/Fragility

Another one in ten (11%) talked about the fragility of life. They used words like "unexpected", "uncertainty" and "less predictable".

The perceived lack of predictability caused many to say they felt a loss of control.

"That it's less predictable than I'd imagine. That things seem inevitable, like graduation ceremonies etc, are incredibly dependent on certain conditions of well-being."

"How uncertain the future is now."

"Everything is just so unexpected."

"Reminds me we aren't as in control as we like to think."

"There is no guarantee for anything now, you just don't know."

"Things can happen when you least expect it and I knew that, but this has been a major reminder."

Importance of health

A similar one in ten respondents (9%) had become more aware of the need to stay healthy and practice good hygiene.

"Always wash your hands and stay clean."

"It's important to take care of yourself and stay healthy."

"Be healthy, stay fit and persevere."

Importance of family

One in ten (9%) said they had refocused on their family and come away with a greater appreciation for all that they provide.

"Family is all that matters most."

"I value spending time with my family more."

"Appreciate the important people in your life."

"How important being with family really is."

"To be more cautious about not spreading germs and not take time with friends or family for granted, not take our freedoms for granted."

The stupidity of others

One in ten respondents (9%) spoke about the selfishness and stupidity of others.

"People are selfish."

"Other people are stupid."

"I'm always right, others don't get it."

"I'm smarter than most."

"Just exactly how stupid some people can be."

"People don't care what authority says."

"People are willing to give up personal freedom and control to the government for temporary safety and security."

Leadership

One in twenty (5%) commented about the leadership or politicians.

"The local community and government have all acted with calm and responsibility (I was pleasantly surprised). Federal and State government, what a disaster, no leadership because no one wants to risk looking bad."

"Not always listen to authority."

"Government is more concerned about the economy than peoples lives."

"Poor leadership."

"Politicians don't really care about people."

Need for social contact

Around one in twenty (4%) had realised the importance of social contact in their lives.

"Humans are very social beings, we need to spend time close to each other."

"The importance of in-person social interaction."

"Interaction and touch is essential for human beings."

"Interaction with others is important, I miss my church."

"We all have to take care of each other, we are connected."

Cautious about other people

A few (3%) expressed concern about the actions of other people.

"You can be screwed by other people's mistakes beyond imagination."

"That we need to be more cautious about other people and places we surround ourselves with."

Being prepared

A few (2%) also made comment about how unprepared society was and the need to be better prepared in future.

"Society was not at all prepared for this type of event."

"It's not fair that I feel safe every day from getting the virus, but others live in fear every day that they will get it because of their job which exposes them to the virus. Don't know the answer, the inequality, but I do

believe all those workers should have the correct protective gear."

Fear and panic

A small number (3%) spoke about people being scared and seeing the fear in others.

"People are scared."

"How people can be put into a panic in such a short time and the affect seems to be infectious."

"How can it change drastically in a very short time."

"80% of the population could not survive in an apocalyptic bunker type situation."

"It taught me the world can change in an instant and that you can't always trust the media and WHO. Information presented as facts is then changed i.e. masks were not useful and now they are mandatory."

Save money

A few (2%) said they'd realised they need to save money in case something happens in the future.

"I've had to ration my food. I need to save more in future."

Other comments

Other one-off comments were about:

"The good work of essential service workers"

"That they could be more productive"

"It's good to slow down"

"Arguments happen when people are cooped up together"

"If you look to the past you will know the future"

"Life can be enjoyed outdoors not just through a phone"

"The America's Health system doesn't work"

"People are resilient"

"Time to fix it and live again".

Chapter 7

Lessons learnt about ourselves (USA)

Respondents were asked what they had learnt about themselves. Their answers fell into 9 categories.

Areas for improvement

The most frequent comments focused on areas they wanted to improve. These were nominated by one in ten respondents (12%). Areas for improvement included:

Be kinder to others
Be more patient
Save money
I can be healthier/a healthier lifestyle
Be more cautious of things around me

Love and trust myself more
Slow down be less busy is good
Wash my hands more
Don't take things for granted/Realise I am blessed.

Resilient, adaptable

Like the West Australian's the American respondents also talked about learning how resilient and strong they were. This was nominated by one in ten respondents (9%)

"I can survive."

"I'm stronger than I thought."

"I can endure anything."

"I can adapt to any situation and I'm very healthy."

"I am not easily made afraid of something I don't have total control of."

Am an introvert

One in twenty (6%) realised they enjoyed social isolating and considered themselves introverts.

"I'm more of an introvert than I thought."

"I found out I'm a hermit naturally."

"I'm an anti-social person after all."

"I've always been a loner so staying home was totally normal for me."

"I'm even more introverted than I thought. This hasn't been too bad. But I am very, very fortunate to have a job where I can work 90% from home and only physically report to my employer when needed."

Need people

Conversely the same proportion (6%) realised they needed people around them.

"I don't do well in isolation."

"I need to be social."

"I'm too sociable to be stuck in the house."

Lack ambition

One in twenty (4%) had come to the realisation that they were lazy, lacked ambition or could achieve more.

"I'm capable of more things. In terms of physical ability and work."

"I'm disappointed by my lack of ambition."

Family

A small number of respondents (3%) said they had come to like spending time with their family.

"I like being with my family more than commuting."

"Our family has grown closer."

Work

A few respondents (3%) talked about their work, with some reassessing their current situation.

"I'm sick of working."

"Realised how much stress work causes me. I find I am less stressed, healthier, and sleeping better during this time."

"I'm fortunate to have a job."

Powerlessness

A few respondents (2%) opened up about feeling powerless.

"That I'm powerless in many ways."

"I'm weak."

"I'm scared I might die."

Other comments

Other one-off comments included:

"I'm a heavy sleeper."

"I need to stay busy/active."

"I'm 'essential."

"I have no self-control around food at work."

"I follow orders well."

"You can't help everyone."

Chapter 8

Other comments about Covid (USA)

Respondents were asked if they wanted to make any other comments about Covid-19 that could help the community. The main additional comments were:

Stay home, especially if you are unwell
Wash your hands, always
Wear a mask
Be considerate/kind to others
Always help those you can
Follow guidelines and listen to medical professionals/listen to government
Don't open things up too soon
Be familiar with your surroundings
Thank you to all who helped to get through this time.

"Being kind and helpful and supportive to others should not only be applied when disaster or other things that affect our county or community but should be something we do on an everyday basis."

Other one-off comments included:

We still need each other, it would be easy to become a recluse but we can't do that
World War 2 Brits knew what they were talking about
We are one world
If you are bored in isolation learn something new
Freedom is a constitutional right
Sometimes the government doesn't know what's best for people
Protesters should be refused medical care if they get sick
Don't eat bats.

"Instead of doing a "fist bump" or touching elbows to greet each other, they can avoid touching altogether and remain 6 feet apart if they acknowledge each other with a "head nod"... no germs will be passed that way."

"This pandemic allows us to manage money better even though under less than average incomes."
"Some people are now gathering to protest the stay-at-home orders, saying our freedom has been taken from us. but that's not the case. This is being done for OUR safety!"

"Investigate Bill Gates, do your own research rather than just believing everything Fox News/ CNN / WHO tells you. Money controls everything. The sickness is real, but follow the money and look who's benefiting the most from it."

"I don't understand why everybody can't get their antibodies tested to see if they have been exposed to the virus. Testing for antibodies is not something new, it's been around for many years. It's not a new test, it's not a new kit someone hasn't develop, it's a simple blood test that can be read in minutes. There are so many people who have had the virus and didn't even know it. Those who test positive could get back to work and get our economy going again and get their lives back again, as far as their income to support their families and prevent small businesses from going bankrupt."

"Need to keep more attentive to other countries biological weapons labs and progress. This also includes right here at home."

Section C: Next Steps

Chapter 9

Next steps

The number one lesson

For me it's been very interesting to hear what others have learnt.

Lets not forget however the number one lesson, the most important learning we can take away from this experience. It was one we learnt early on, right at the start of the pandemic.

One that shocked us in its simplicity.

One that taught us so much about humanity and its many sides.

"Never, ever, ever let your toilet paper supply run down to less than two months' worth."

You can thank me later. Seriously though, the main thing I learnt was the value of friendship. I was absolutely blown away by the people who offered help at the first sight of a potential problem. In some respect Covid-19 reinstated my love of humanity.

What have you learnt about yourself?

What will you do differently?

How was your takeout different?

What should we keep in life after Covid-19? We'll be writing about that in the next book.

KEY AREAS

Consumer psychology/branding consultant, Business owner
Consumer advocate (Disability, Carers), Board member
Author, Freelance writer, Speaker

BACKGROUND

Glennys's passion for people saw her qualify as a psychologist in the 1980s and then spend over 20 years studying consumer behaviour.

Her first job after university was as Promotions Officer with the Australian Red Cross, where she spent three years travelling around Western Australia to places like Useless Loop. While at the Australian Red Cross she was responsible for the *Youth News* magazine, which went out to all West Australian schools.

She then spent 8 years at HBF establishing and managing the Market Research Department which is still in existence today. During that time she helped develop and manage the Ted campaign, a highly successful brand campaign that generated awareness figures similar to Coca Cola.

In 2000 she opened an independent consumer psychology consultancy, *The Customers' Voice*, through which she has helped numerous blue-chip clients develop marketing plans, advertising campaigns and new products. Her clients include the Australian Defence Force, Chevron, ECU, Telstra/Telecom, and Woolworths to name a few. She's also delved into a wide range of social issues including - investigating drug/alcohol related problems during the America's Cup; the *Speed Catches Up With You* drug campaign and a national study into family/domestic violence/sexual assault. All of which has enabled her to interact with a diverse range of people.

In 2007 she published her first book, *50 Ways To Grieve Your Lover,* after the passing of her partner. This was taken up by the likes of the Australian Red Cross, Solaris Care and others. It was also used by counsellors working in the Victorian Bush Fires and New Zealand Pike Mine Disaster.

In 2008 she wrote her first piece of fiction *'A Whales Tale'*, which won first prize in the Stirling Literary Awards. This led to more freelance writing gigs including a monthly column in *Swan Magazine* (since 2015) and regular gigs with *Arts Australia, Visit Perth City, So Perth, The Weekly Review* (Melbourne), *Divine* (Disability) and *ABC Ramp It Up* to name a few.

Due to the success of her book, in 2008 she also started a blog called *The Ponder Room* which attracted an international audience across 20+ countries after just six months.

In 2012 she wrote her second book *Me Time: 100 Ways To Get Guilt Free Me Time,* after watching several workaholic friends get sick or take their life. The book was heralded by new mums and busy executives. A presentation on this topic won a People's Choice Award. For more books by Glennys see below.

She currently spreads her time between freelance research projects, writing jobs and sitting on several advisory Boards.

She also conducts workshops, speaking engagements and personal mentoring sessions covering topics such as Personal Branding, Consumer Psychology, Writing Your First Book, Overcoming Grief and Gaining Guilt Free Me Time.

RECOGNITION

Australia Day City of Perth Community **Citizen Of The Year 2020** nominee.

Consumer Protection Award: Rona Okely Award 2019 winner (For an individual who has given their time, energy and experience to the betterment of others). This was based on her years spent researching and advocating for W.A. consumers across a wide range of issues. It also acknowledged her time spent volunteering on the MSWA Board, the Carers Advisory Council as well as the Consumer Protection's Consumer Advisory Committee.

People's Choice Award at the Australian Market and Social Research Society Conference 2013. For a presentation based on her second book *Me Time 100 Strategies For Guilt Free Me Time.*

Telstra Business Women's Award 2012 - nominee

Profiled by US internet and marketing guru Seth Godin, in his book *True Stories of People Poking the Box and Making a Difference* (2011). Her nomination was due to the impact of *50 Ways To Grieve Your Lover*

Rigby Award 2010. For services to cartooning due to her work on the *Michael Collins Caricature Award,* which was established to honour her partner and raised funds for the Heart Foundation. The award ran for four years.

For more information go to Website
www.glennysmarsdon.com
Email: admin (at) glennysmarsdon (dot) com

Books by the author

BOOKS BY Glennys Marsdon

1. *Covid-19: 40 Lessons Learnt about Life and Ourselves (2020) – Western Australia edition*
2. *Covid-19: 2- Lessons Learnt about Life and Ourselves (2020) – USA edition*
3. *25 Simple Canned Tuna Recipes (2020)*
4. *30 Tips To Successfully Work From Home (2020)*
5. *Impact: 45 Tips To Help You Get Involved And Make A Difference (2020)*
6. *Wit and Wisdom (2019)*
7. *15 Frequently Asked Questions to Consider Before Writing an eBook (2019)*
8. *Freelance Life: An Action Plan To Help You Become A Successful Six Figure Freelancer (2016)*
9. *Me Time: 100 Strategies For Guilt Free Me Time. (2012)*
10. *50 Ways To Grieve Your Lover: 100 Tips Gaining Back Control (2007)*
11. *A Bouquet of Love (Anthology)*
12. *All Wrapped Up (Anthology)*

Guest speaking. Workshops. Consulting

GUEST SPEAKING. WORKSHOPS

With 20+ years spent facilitating groups, Glennys is a sought-after speaker and moderator on the following topics. To book her email admin (at) glennysmarsdon (dot) com.

Personal Development e.g. Health and Mental Health:
How to make an impact
How to develop a Personal Brand
Overcoming Grief
Gaining back control
How to get guilt free Me Time

Business:
How to write and publish an eBook
How to become a successful Freelancer
Branding and Marketing Tips for Business
Consumer Psychology e.g. Why We Do What We Do

CONSULTING AND MENTORING

As discussed earlier, Glennys has worked as a freelance consultant for 20+ years through her business The Customers' Voice (TCV), through which she has helped numerous blue-chip clients develop:

Marketing plans and advertising campaigns
New products
Key Performance Indications
Customer Satisfaction measures
Employee surveys
Social issues e.g. domestic violence

She is also available for one on one mentoring sessions. To book her email admin (at) glennysmarsdon (dot) com.

www.ingramcontent.com/pod-product-compliance
Lightning Source LLC
Chambersburg PA
CBHW072154020426
42334CB00018B/2010